EAT RIGHT, BURN CALORIES

The Essential Cookbook for Effective and Effortless Weight Loss with Delicious, Flavorful and Nourishing Recipes

DR HELENA M. OLIVIA

Copyright Page

TABLE OF CONTENTS

UNDERSTANDING THE CONCEPT OF ZERO POINT FOOD

Zero Point foods is designed to support a balanced and sustainable approach to healthy eating, focusing on nutrient-dense foods while allowing for flexibility and enjoyment in food choices. Here's a breakdown of the concept and how it works:

1. **Nutrient-rich foods**: Zero Point foods typically include fruits, vegetables, lean proteins, and some whole grains. These foods are chosen because they tend to be lower in calories while providing essential nutrients like vitamins, minerals, fiber, and protein.

- **Freedom to eat**: When a food is designated as a Zero Point food, it means you can eat it without having to track or count its SmartPoints value. This provides a sense of freedom and flexibility in meal planning and allows you to focus on eating nutritious foods that help you feel satisfied and energized.

- **Encourages healthy choices**: By emphasizing Zero Point foods, the program encourages participants to base their meals around these healthier options.

- This can help improve overall dietary patterns by increasing intake of fruits, vegetables, and lean proteins, which are associated with numerous health benefits, including weight management, improved digestion, and reduced risk of chronic diseases.

- **Portion control:** While Zero Point foods are free to eat, portion control is still important. Eating unlimited quantities of even healthy foods can lead to overconsumption of calories, which may hinder weight loss or maintenance goals. The program encourages mindful eating and listening to hunger and fullness cues to help regulate portion sizes.

- **Flexibility:** Although Zero Point foods are encouraged, the program also allows for flexibility and moderation. Participants still have a daily Smart Points budget that can be used for foods that are not Zero Point, such as treats or higher-calorie items. This flexibility makes the program sustainable and adaptable to individual preferences and lifestyles.

HOW ZERO POINT FOODS CONTRIBUTE TO A HEALTHY LIFESTYLE

Zero-point foods contribute to a healthy lifestyle by providing essential nutrients, supporting weight management, reducing the risk of chronic diseases, boosting immune function, promoting healthy aging, improving mood and mental health, increasing energy levels, supporting environmental sustainability, and being budget-friendly.

- **Nutrient Density:** Many zero-point foods are rich in essential nutrients such as vitamins, minerals, and antioxidants.
- **Calorie Control:** Since zero-point foods are low in calories, they can help with calorie control and weight management. They allow you to fill up on nutritious options without consuming excessive calories, making it easier to maintain a healthy weight.
- **Hydration:** Many zero-point foods, especially fruits and vegetables, have high water content, which contributes to hydration.
- **Blood Sugar Control:** Foods like non-starchy vegetables and lean proteins have minimal impact on blood sugar levels, which is beneficial for individuals with diabetes or those looking to stabilize their blood sugar levels.

- **Heart Health:** Many zero-point foods, such as fruits, vegetables, and lean proteins, are beneficial for heart health due to their low saturated fat and cholesterol content.
- **Digestive Health:** The fiber found in many zero-point foods supports digestive health by promoting regular bowel movements and preventing constipation.
- **Reduced Risk of Chronic Diseases:** A diet rich in zero-point foods, particularly fruits and vegetables, has been linked to a reduced risk of chronic diseases such as certain cancers, cardiovascular disease, and diabetes.
- **Improved Immune Function:** Many zero-point foods, especially fruits and vegetables, are rich in vitamins A, C, and E, as well as other nutrients that support immune function.

SHOPPING FOR ZERO POINT FOODS

Shopping for zero point foods typically involves selecting foods that are low in calories and high in nutrients, as they are designated as "zero points" on certain weight loss programs. Here's a list of common zero point foods:

- **Fruits:** *Apples, Bananas, Berries (strawberries, blueberries, raspberries, blackberries), Oranges, Grapefruit, Peaches, Pears, Plums, Kiwi, Melons (watermelon, cantaloupe, honeydew), Grapes, Pineapple, Mango, Cherries etc.*

- **Vegetables:** *Spinach, Kale, Lettuce (all varieties), Arugula, Swiss chard, Collard greens, Mustard greens, Turnip greens, Beet greens, Broccoli, Cauliflower, Carrots, Bell peppers (all colors), Cucumbers, Tomatoes, Celery, Radishes, Green beans, Snap peas, Asparagus, Zucchini, Summer squash, Eggplant, Mushrooms, Onions, Garlic, Leeks, Scallions, Brussels sprouts, Cabbage (green, red, Napa), Spaghetti squash, Butternut squash, Acorn squash, Pumpkin*

- **Lean proteins:** *Skinless chicken breast, turkey breast, tofu, fish (such as salmon or cod), shellfish (like shrimp or crab), eggs, plain Greek yogurt (non-fat), cottage cheese (non-fat), beans, lentils, etc.*

- **Whole grains:** *Quinoa, brown rice, oats, barley, whole wheat pasta, etc.*

- **Non-starchy vegetables:** *Asparagus, cauliflower, zucchini, cabbage, kale, Brussels sprouts, etc.*

- **Condiments and seasonings:** *Herbs, spices, vinegar, mustard, hot sauce, salsa, Lemon juice, Lime juice, Pickles (dill, gherkins, etc.), Capers, Unsweetened almond milk, Unsweetened coconut milk, Unsweetened soy milk etc.*

When shopping for zero point foods, focus on fresh produce, lean proteins, and whole grains. Avoid processed foods and those high in added sugars and fats. It's also essential to read labels carefully, as some foods may seem healthy but can contain hidden sugars or unhealthy fats. Buying in bulk and planning meals ahead of time can help you incorporate these zero point foods into your diet effectively.

WHAT TO AVOID WHEN SHOPPING FOR ZERO POINT FOODS

When shopping for Zero Point Foods, which are often associated with weight loss and healthy eating plans, it's essential to be mindful of a few key considerations to ensure you're making the healthiest choices possible. Here are some things to avoid:

- **Processed Foods**: While some processed foods may still be considered Zero Point Foods due to their low-calorie content, they may lack essential nutrients and contain additives, preservatives, and excessive sodium or sugar.
- **Added Sugars:** Even if a food is listed as a Zero Point Food, it's crucial to check the label for added sugars. High sugar intake can lead to various health issues, including weight gain, diabetes, and heart disease.
- **Highly Caloric Foods:** While Zero Point Foods are meant to be low in calories, some naturally calorie-dense foods, like nuts and avocados, are not included in this category. While they are healthy in moderation, consuming them excessively could hinder weight loss efforts.

- **Overindulgence:** Just because a food is labeled as Zero Points doesn't mean you should consume unlimited quantities of it. Portion control is still important for overall health and weight management.

- **Ignoring All Other Nutritional Information:** While a food may be Zero Points, it's essential to consider its overall nutritional value. For example, a food may be low in calories but high in unhealthy fats or lacking in essential vitamins and minerals.

VEGETABLE HASH WITH POACHED EGGS

PREP	**COOK**	**YIELDS**	**SERVING SIZE**
10 Mins	15 Mins	4 Servings	1/4

INGREDIENTS

- 1 cup diced zucchini
- 1 cup diced bell peppers (any color)
- 1 cup diced mushrooms
- 1 cup diced tomatoes
- 1/2 cup diced onions
- 2 cloves garlic, minced
- Salt and pepper to taste
- Cooking spray
- 4 large eggs
- Chopped parsley for garnish (optional)

DIRECTIONS

- In a non-stick skillet, heat cooking spray over medium heat.
- Add onions and garlic to the skillet and sauté for 2-3 minutes until they begin to soften.
- Add zucchini, bell peppers, mushrooms, and tomatoes to the skillet. Season with salt and pepper. Cook, stirring occasionally, for about 8-10 minutes until vegetables are tender.
- While the vegetables are cooking, poach the eggs. Bring a pot of water to a gentle simmer. Crack eggs, one at a time, into a small bowl or ramekin.

- Calories: 70kcal
- Total Fat: 2g
- Saturated Fat: 0.5g
- Cholesterol: 186mg
- Sodium: 50mg
- Carbohydrates: 8g
- Dietary Fiber: 2g
- Sugars: 4g
- Protein: 6g

DIRECTIONS

- Carefully slide each egg into the simmering water. Cook for about 3-4 minutes for a soft poached egg.
- Once the vegetables are cooked and the eggs are poached, divide the vegetable hash evenly among four plates.
- Carefully remove poached eggs from the water with a slotted spoon and place one on top of each serving of vegetable hash.
- Garnish with chopped parsley if desired, and serve immediately.

GARLIC CHILLED EDAMAME

PREP
5 Mins

COOK
5 Mins

YIELDS
4 Servings

SERVING SIZE
1/2

INGREDIENTS

- 2 cups shelled edamame
- 2 cloves garlic, minced
- 2 tablespoons chopped fresh cilantro
- 2 tablespoons rice vinegar
- 1 tablespoon soy sauce
- 1 teaspoon sesame oil
- Salt and pepper to taste
- Optional: red pepper flakes for heat

DIRECTIONS

- Bring a pot of water to a boil. Add the shelled edamame and cook for about 3-4 minutes, or until tender. Drain and rinse under cold water to stop the cooking process.
- In a small bowl, mix together minced garlic, chopped cilantro, rice vinegar, soy sauce, sesame oil, salt, pepper, and red pepper flakes if desired.
- In a large mixing bowl, toss the cooked and cooled edamame with the prepared dressing until evenly coated.
- Cover the bowl and refrigerate the dressed edamame for at least 30 minutes to allow the flavors to meld together.

NUTRITIONAL FACTS (PER SERVING)

- Calories: 85kcal
- Total Fat: 3g
- Saturated Fat: 0.5g
- Cholesterol: 0mg
- Sodium: 148mg
- Carbohydrates: 7g
- Dietary Fiber: 3g
- Sugars: 1g
- Protein: 7g

DIRECTIONS

- Once chilled, serve the garlic chilled edamame as a refreshing and healthy snack or side dish.

CABBAGE AND CARROT SLAW WITH APPLE CIDER VINEGAR DRESSING

PREP
10 Mins

COOK
40 Mins

YIELDS
4 Servings

SERVING SIZE
1 cup

INGREDIENTS

- 4 cups shredded green cabbage
- 1 cup shredded carrots
- 2 tablespoons apple cider vinegar
- 1 tablespoon olive oil
- 1 teaspoon honey (optional)
- Salt and pepper to taste

DIRECTIONS

- In a large bowl, combine the shredded cabbage and carrots.
- In a small bowl, whisk together the apple cider vinegar, olive oil, honey (if using), salt, and pepper to make the dressing.
- Pour the dressing over the cabbage and carrot mixture, tossing well to coat evenly.
- Cover the bowl and refrigerate for at least 30 minutes before serving to allow the flavors to meld.

NUTRITIONAL FACTS (PER SERVING)

- Calories: 50kcal
- Total Fat: 3g
- Saturated Fat: <1g
- Cholesterol: 0mg
- Sodium: 30mg
- Carbohydrates: 6g
- Dietary Fiber: 2g
- Sugars: 3g
- Protein: 1g

CHILI CHICKEN MUSHROOM BUN BURGERS

PREP	**COOK**	**YIELDS**	**SERVING SIZE**
10 Mins	15 Mins	4 Servings	1

INGREDIENTS

- 1 lb ground chicken breast
- 1 cup mushrooms, finely chopped
- 1 small onion, finely chopped
- 2 cloves garlic, minced
- 1 tablespoon chili powder
- 1 teaspoon cumin
- Salt and pepper to taste
- Lettuce leaves (for buns)

DIRECTIONS

- In a mixing bowl, combine ground chicken, mushrooms, onion, garlic, chili powder, cumin, salt, and pepper. Mix until well combined.
- Divide the mixture into equal portions and shape them into burger patties.
- Preheat a non-stick skillet over medium heat. Cook the patties for about 5-7 minutes on each side, or until fully cooked through.
- Once cooked, remove from heat and let them rest for a few minutes.
- To assemble the burgers, place a lettuce leaf on a plate, then place a cooked patty on top of the lettuce.

NUTRITIONAL FACTS (PER SERVING)

- Calories: 150kcal
- Total Fat: 6g
- Saturated Fat: 1.5g
- Trans Fat: 0g
- Cholesterol: 85mg
- Sodium: 280mg
- Carbohydrates: 4g
- Dietary Fiber: 1g
- Sugars: 1g
- Protein: 20g

DIRECTIONS

- Add any additional toppings or condiments of your choice.
- Serve immediately and enjoy!

ITALIAN VEGETABLE SOUP

PREP
10 Mins

COOK
25 Mins

YIELDS
6 Servings

SERVING SIZE
1 cup

INGREDIENTS

- 1 onion, diced
- 2 cloves garlic, minced
- 2 carrots, diced
- 2 celery stalks, diced
- 1 zucchini, diced
- 1 yellow squash, diced
- 1 can (14.5 oz) diced tomatoes, with juices
- 4 cups fat-free vegetable broth
- 1 teaspoon dried oregano
- 1 teaspoon dried basil
- Salt and pepper to taste
- Chopped fresh parsley for garnish (optional)

DIRECTIONS

- In a large pot, sauté the onion and garlic over medium heat until softened.
- Add carrots and celery, and cook for another 2-3 minutes.
- Stir in zucchini and yellow squash, cooking for an additional 2 minutes.
- Pour in diced tomatoes with their juices and vegetable broth. Bring to a simmer.
- Add dried oregano, dried basil, salt, and pepper. Stir well.
- Let the soup simmer for about 20-25 minutes until the vegetables are tender.
- Taste and adjust seasoning if needed.
- Serve hot, garnished with chopped parsley if desired.

NUTRITIONAL FACTS (PER SERVING)

- Calories: 50kcal
- Total Fat: 0g
- Saturated Fat: 0g
- Cholesterol: 0mg
- Sodium: 480mg
- Carbohydrates: 11g
- Dietary Fiber: 3g
- Sugars: 5g
- Protein: 2g

CAULIFLOWER PILAF

PREP
10 Mins

COOK
15 Mins

YIELDS
4 Servings

SERVING SIZE
1/4

INGREDIENTS

- 1 medium head cauliflower, grated
- 1 small onion, finely chopped
- 2 cloves garlic, minced
- 1 cup diced bell peppers (any color)
- 1 cup diced tomatoes
- 1 teaspoon ground cumin
- 1 teaspoon paprika
- Salt and pepper to taste
- Fresh cilantro or parsley for garnish (optional)

DIRECTIONS

- Heat a large non-stick skillet over medium heat. Add the chopped onion and garlic. Cook until softened, about 2-3 minutes.
- Add the grated cauliflower to the skillet. Cook, stirring occasionally, until the cauliflower begins to soften, about 5-7 minutes.
- Stir in the diced bell peppers and tomatoes. Cook for an additional 5 minutes, or until the vegetables are tender.
- Sprinkle the ground cumin and paprika over the cauliflower mixture. Season with salt and pepper to taste. Stir well to combine.
- Cook for another 2-3 minutes, allowing the flavors to meld together.

NUTRITIONAL FACTS (PER SERVING)

- Calories: 50kcal
- Total Fat: 0g
- Saturated Fat: 0g
- Cholesterol: 0mg
- Sodium: 80mg
- Carbohydrates: 10g
- Dietary Fiber: 4g
- Sugars: 5g
- Protein: 3g

DIRECTIONS

- Remove from heat and garnish with fresh cilantro or parsley if desired. Serve hot.

ZOODLE PASTA PRIMAVERA

PREP	**COOK**	**YIELDS**	**SERVING SIZE**
10 Mins	10 Mins	4 Servings	1/4

INGREDIENTS

- 4 medium zucchinis, spiralized
- 1 cup cherry tomatoes, halved
- 1 cup sliced bell peppers (any color)
- 1 cup sliced mushrooms
- 1 small onion, thinly sliced
- 2 cloves garlic, minced
- 1 tablespoon olive oil
- 1 teaspoon Italian seasoning
- Salt and pepper to taste
- Optional: red pepper flakes for heat
- Fresh basil leaves for garnish (optional)

DIRECTIONS

- Spiralize the zucchinis and set aside. Slice all the vegetables as instructed.
- Heat olive oil in a large skillet over medium heat. Add minced garlic and sliced onion. Sauté until the onion becomes translucent, about 2-3 minutes.
- Add bell peppers and mushrooms to the skillet. Cook for another 3-4 minutes until they start to soften.
- Add cherry tomatoes, Italian seasoning, salt, pepper, and red pepper flakes if desired. Cook for an additional 2-3 minutes until the tomatoes start to soften and release their juices.

NUTRITIONAL FACTS (PER SERVING)

- Calories: 55kcal
- Total Fat: 3g
- Saturated Fat: 0.5g
- Trans Fat: 0g
- Cholesterol: 0mg
- Sodium: 10mg
- Carbohydrates: 7g
- Dietary Fiber: 2g
- Sugars: 4g
- Protein: 2g

DIRECTIONS

- Add the spiralized zucchini to the skillet. Toss everything together gently and cook for 2-3 minutes until the zoodles are heated through but still slightly crisp.
- Serve: Remove from heat and garnish with fresh basil leaves if desired.

CAULIFLOWER CRUST MINI PIZZAS WITH TOMATO AND BASIL

PREP
15 Mins

COOK
30 Mins

YIELDS
4 Servings

SERVING SIZE
1

INGREDIENTS

- 2 cups cauliflower rice
- 1 egg
- 1/2 teaspoon garlic powder
- 1/2 teaspoon onion powder
- Salt and pepper to taste
- Tomato sauce (look for sugar-free or low-sugar options)
- Fresh basil leaves, chopped
- Optional toppings: sliced cherry tomatoes, sliced olives, diced bell peppers, etc.

DIRECTIONS

- Preheat your oven to 400°F (200°C). Line a baking sheet with parchment paper or lightly grease it.
- In a microwave-safe bowl, microwave the cauliflower rice for 5-6 minutes or until tender. Allow it to cool slightly.
- Once the cauliflower rice has cooled, transfer it to a clean kitchen towel and squeeze out as much moisture as possible.
- In a mixing bowl, combine the cauliflower rice, egg, garlic powder, onion powder, salt, and pepper. Mix well to form a dough.

NUTRITIONAL FACTS (PER SERVING)

- Calories: 50kcal
- Fat: 1g
- Carbohydrates: 5g
- Protein: 3g
- Fiber: 2g
- Sugar: 2g

DIRECTIONS

- Divide the dough into small portions and shape them into mini pizza crusts on the prepared baking sheet.
- Bake the cauliflower crusts in the preheated oven for 20-25 minutes or until they are firm and golden brown.
- Remove the crusts from the oven and let them cool slightly.
- Once cooled, top each crust with a spoonful of tomato sauce and sprinkle with chopped basil leaves.
- Add any additional toppings of your choice.
- Return the mini pizzas to the oven and bake for an additional 5-10 minutes, or until the toppings are heated through.
- Serve hot and enjoy!

MUSHROOM LENTIL SLICE

PREP
15 Mins

COOK
30 Mins

YIELDS
6 Servings

SERVING SIZE
1/6

INGREDIENTS

- 1 cup cooked lentils
- 2 cups sliced mushrooms
- 1 small onion, diced
- 2 cloves garlic, minced
- 1/2 cup rolled oats
- 2 tablespoons nutritional yeast
- 1 teaspoon dried thyme
- Salt and pepper to taste
- Cooking spray

DIRECTIONS

- Preheat your oven to 375°F (190°C).
- In a non-stick skillet, sauté the onions and garlic until translucent, about 5 minutes.
- Add the sliced mushrooms to the skillet and cook until they release their moisture and become tender, about 7-8 minutes.
- In a large mixing bowl, combine the cooked lentils, sautéed mushrooms, onion, garlic, rolled oats, nutritional yeast, dried thyme, salt, and pepper. Mix well to combine.
- Spray a baking dish with cooking spray and spread the lentil mixture evenly into the dish.

NUTRITIONAL FACTS (PER SERVING)

- Calories: 110kcal
- Protein: 7g
- Carbohydrates: 20g
- Fat: 1g
- Fiber: 5g

DIRECTIONS

- Bake in the preheated oven for 25-30 minutes or until the slice is set and lightly golden on top.
- Allow the slice to cool slightly before slicing into portions.

VEGAN BEAN AND TOMATO RAGU

PREP
10 Mins

COOK
20 Mins

YIELDS
4 Servings

SERVING SIZE
1

INGREDIENTS

- 1 can (15 oz) kidney beans, drained and rinsed
- 1 can (15 oz) cannellini beans, drained and rinsed
- 1 can (15 oz) black beans, drained and rinsed
- 1 can (15 oz) diced tomatoes
- 1 onion, diced
- 2 cloves garlic, minced
- 1 teaspoon dried oregano
- 1 teaspoon dried basil
- 1 teaspoon paprika
- Salt and pepper to taste
- Fresh parsley, chopped (for garnish)

DIRECTIONS

- In a large skillet or saucepan, sauté the diced onion and minced garlic until softened, about 3-5 minutes.
- Add the diced tomatoes (undrained) to the skillet along with the drained and rinsed beans.
- Stir in the dried oregano, dried basil, paprika, salt, and pepper.
- Bring the mixture to a simmer over medium heat and let it cook for about 15 minutes, stirring occasionally, until the flavors meld together and the sauce thickens slightly.
- Taste and adjust seasoning if needed.
- Serve the vegan bean and tomato ragu hot, garnished with fresh parsley if desired.

NUTRITIONAL FACTS (PER SERVING)

- Calories: 215kcal
- Total Fat: 1g
- Saturated Fat: 0g
- Cholesterol: 0mg
- Sodium: 455mg
- Carbohydrates: 39g
- Dietary Fiber: 13g
- Sugars: 5g
- Protein: 13g

CHINESE CHICKEN RISSOLES

PREP
10 Mins

COOK
25 Mins

YIELDS
4 Servings

SERVING SIZE
3

INGREDIENTS

- 1 pound ground chicken breast
- 2 cloves garlic, minced
- 2 tablespoons low-sodium soy sauce
- 2 teaspoons grated fresh ginger
- 1/4 cup chopped scallions
- 1/4 cup chopped water chestnuts
- 1/4 cup chopped cilantro
- 1/2 teaspoon salt
- 1/4 teaspoon black pepper
- Cooking spray

DIRECTIONS

- Preheat your oven to 375°F (190°C).
- In a large bowl, combine ground chicken, garlic, soy sauce, ginger, scallions, water chestnuts, cilantro, salt, and pepper. Mix well to combine.
- Form the mixture into 12 equal-sized rissoles and place them on a baking sheet lined with parchment paper.
- Lightly spray the rissoles with cooking spray.
- Bake in the preheated oven for 20-25 minutes, or until cooked through and golden brown.

NUTRITIONAL FACTS (PER SERVING)

- Calories: 150kcal
- Total Fat: 3g
- Saturated Fat: 0.5g
- Trans Fat: 0g
- Cholesterol: 75mg
- Sodium: 550mg
- Carbohydrates: 3g
- Dietary Fiber: 1g
- Sugars: 0g
- Protein: 25g

DIRECTIONS

- Serve hot, garnished with fresh cilantro or parsley if desired.

TURKEY TIKKA MASALA WITH CAULIFLOWER RICE

PREP	**COOK**	**YIELDS**	**SERVING SIZE**
10 Mins	20 Mins	4 Servings	1 cup

INGREDIENTS

- 1 lb lean ground turkey
- 1 onion, diced
- 3 cloves garlic, minced
- 1 tablespoon ginger, grated
- 1 tablespoon tomato paste
- 1 tablespoon garam masala
- 1 teaspoon ground cumin
- 1 teaspoon ground coriander
- 1 teaspoon paprika
- 1/2 teaspoon turmeric
- 1/2 teaspoon cayenne pepper (adjust to taste)
- 1 cup fat-free Greek yogurt
- 1 cup chicken or vegetable broth
- Salt and pepper to taste
- Fresh cilantro, chopped (for garnish)
- 1 head cauliflower, riced (or store-bought cauliflower rice)

DIRECTIONS

- In a large skillet over medium heat, cook the ground turkey until browned and cooked through, breaking it apart with a spoon as it cooks. Remove turkey from skillet and set aside.
- In the same skillet, add diced onion and cook until softened, about 5 minutes. Add minced garlic and grated ginger, cook for another minute until fragrant.
- Stir in tomato paste, garam masala, cumin, coriander, paprika, turmeric, and cayenne pepper. Cook for 1-2 minutes until spices are toasted and fragrant.
- Return the cooked turkey to the skillet.

NUTRITIONAL FACTS (PER SERVING)

- Calories: 200kcal
- Protein: 25g
- Carbohydrates: 9g
- Fat: 7g
- Fiber: 3g

DIRECTIONS

- Stir in Greek yogurt and chicken or vegetable broth. Simmer for 10-15 minutes until the sauce has thickened slightly and flavors have melded together. Season with salt and pepper to taste.
- While the tikka masala is simmering, prepare the cauliflower rice by pulsing cauliflower florets in a food processor until they resemble rice grains.
- Serve the turkey tikka masala over cauliflower rice, garnished with chopped cilantro.

CURRIED RED LENTIL CHICKPEA STEW

PREP	**COOK**	**YIELDS**	**SERVING SIZE**
10 Mins	25 Mins	6 Servings	1

INGREDIENTS

- 1 cup dry red lentils
- 1 can (15 oz) chickpeas, drained and rinsed
- 1 onion, diced
- 2 cloves garlic, minced
- 1 can (14.5 oz) diced tomatoes
- 3 cups vegetable broth
- 1 tablespoon curry powder
- 1 teaspoon ground cumin
- 1 teaspoon ground turmeric
- 1/2 teaspoon ground ginger
- Salt and pepper to taste
- Fresh cilantro for garnish (optional)

DIRECTIONS

- In a large pot, sauté the diced onion and minced garlic over medium heat until softened.
- Add the curry powder, ground cumin, ground turmeric, and ground ginger to the pot, stirring for about 1 minute until fragrant.
- Add the dry red lentils, chickpeas, diced tomatoes, and vegetable broth to the pot. Stir well to combine.
- Bring the stew to a boil, then reduce the heat to low and let it simmer for about 20-25 minutes, or until the lentils are tender, stirring occasionally.
- Season the stew with salt and pepper to taste.
- Serve the stew hot, garnished with fresh cilantro if desired.

NUTRITIONAL FACTS (PER SERVING)

- Calories: 180kcal
- Total Fat: 1g
- Saturated Fat: 0g
- Cholesterol: 0mg
- Sodium: 420mg
- Carbohydrates: 34g
- Dietary Fiber: 10g
- Sugars: 5g
- Protein: 11g

SPAGHETTI SQUASH WITH TOMATO AND GARLIC SAUCE

PREP	**COOK**	**YIELDS**	**SERVING SIZE**
10 Mins	40 Mins	4 Servings	1/4 cup

INGREDIENTS

- 1 medium spaghetti squash
- 2 cups tomato sauce (ensure it's zero points)
- 2 cloves garlic, minced
- Salt and pepper to taste
- Optional: chopped fresh basil or parsley for garnish

DIRECTIONS

- Preheat your oven to 375°F (190°C).
- Cut the spaghetti squash in half lengthwise and scoop out the seeds.
- Place the squash halves cut side down on a baking sheet lined with parchment paper.
- Bake for 30-40 minutes, or until the squash is tender and easily pierced with a fork.
- While the squash is baking, prepare the sauce. In a saucepan, sauté the minced garlic until fragrant.
- Add the tomato sauce to the saucepan and heat through. Season with salt and pepper to taste.
- Once the squash is done, use a fork to scrape the flesh into spaghetti-like strands.

NUTRITIONAL FACTS (PER SERVING)

- Calories: 80kcal
- Total Fat: 0g
- Saturated Fat: 0g
- Cholesterol: 0mg
- Sodium: 300mg
- Carbohydrates: 18g
- Dietary Fiber: 4g
- Sugars: 8g
- Protein: 2g

DIRECTIONS

- Serve the spaghetti squash topped with the tomato and garlic sauce.
- Garnish with chopped fresh basil or parsley if desired.

SOUFFLE OMELET WITH STRAWBERRIES

PREP
5 Mins

COOK
10 Mins

YIELDS
1 Serving

SERVING SIZE
1

INGREDIENTS

- 3 large egg whites
- 1/4 teaspoon cream of tartar
- 1/4 cup sliced strawberries
- 1 teaspoon zero-calorie sweetener (optional)
- Cooking spray

DIRECTIONS

- Preheat your oven to 375°F (190°C).
- Separate the egg whites from the yolks. Place the egg whites in a mixing bowl and add the cream of tartar.
- Using an electric mixer, beat the egg whites until stiff peaks form.
- Gently fold in the sliced strawberries and zero-calorie sweetener, if using.
- Lightly coat a small oven-safe skillet with cooking spray and place it over medium heat.
- Pour the egg white mixture into the skillet and spread it evenly.
- Cook for 2-3 minutes until the bottom is set.

**NUTRITIONAL FACTS
(PER SERVING)**

- Calories: 60kcal
- Protein: 11g
- Carbohydrates: 3g
- Fat: 0g
- Fiber: 1g
- Sugar: 2g
- Sodium: 176mg

DIRECTIONS

- Transfer the skillet to the preheated oven and bake for an additional 5-7 minutes, or until the omelet is puffed up and lightly golden.
- Carefully remove from the oven and serve immediately.

GRILLED STONE FRUIT

| **PREP**
5 Mins | **COOK**
7 Mins | **YIELDS**
8 Servings | **SERVING SIZE**
1/2 |

INGREDIENTS

- 4 stone fruits (such as peaches, plums, nectarines), halved and pitted
- Cooking spray (preferably olive oil spray)
- Optional: pinch of cinnamon or a drizzle of honey (adjust points if used)

DIRECTIONS

- Preheat your grill to medium-high heat.
- Lightly coat the cut side of each fruit half with cooking spray.
- Place the fruit halves, cut side down, onto the preheated grill.
- Grill for about 3-4 minutes or until grill marks form and the fruit softens slightly. Flip and grill for an additional 2-3 minutes.
- Remove from the grill and serve immediately.
- Optionally, sprinkle with a pinch of cinnamon or drizzle with honey if desired.

NUTRITIONAL FACTS (PER SERVING)

- Calories: 35kcal
- Total Fat: 0g
- Saturated Fat: 0g
- Cholesterol: 0mg
- Sodium: 0mg
- Carbohydrate: 9g
- Dietary Fiber: 1g
- Sugars: 8g
- Protein: 1g

BANANA BREAD MUFFINS

PREP	**COOK**	**YIELDS**	**SERVING SIZE**
10 Mins	25 Mins	12 Servings	1

INGREDIENTS

- 2 ripe bananas, mashed
- 1 cup unsweetened applesauce
- 1 teaspoon vanilla extract
- 1 1/2 cups self-rising flour

DIRECTIONS

- Preheat your oven to 350°F (175°C). Line a muffin tin with paper liners or spray with non-stick cooking spray.
- In a mixing bowl, combine mashed bananas, applesauce, and vanilla extract. Mix well.
- Gradually add self-rising flour to the banana mixture, stirring until just combined. Be careful not to overmix.
- Pour the batter evenly into the prepared muffin tin, filling each cup about 3/4 full.
- Bake in the preheated oven for 20-25 minutes, or until a toothpick inserted into the center of a muffin comes out clean.

NUTRITIONAL FACTS (PER SERVING)

- Calories: 70kcal
- Total Fat: 0g
- Saturated Fat: 0g
- Cholesterol: 0mg
- Sodium: 100mg
- Carbohydrates: 16g
- Dietary Fiber: 1g
- Sugars: 5g
- Protein: 1g

DIRECTIONS

- Allow muffins to cool in the tin for a few minutes before transferring to a wire rack to cool completely.

AVOCADO AND PRAWN COCKTAIL WITH MARIE ROSE SAUCE

<table>
<tr><td>PREP
10 Mins</td><td>COOK
0 Mins</td><td>YIELDS
2 Servings</td><td>SERVING SIZE
1/2</td></tr>
</table>

INGREDIENTS

- 200g cooked prawns, peeled and deveined
- 1 ripe avocado, diced
- 2 tablespoons fat-free Greek yogurt
- 2 tablespoons tomato ketchup (use sugar-free for zero points)
- 1 teaspoon Worcestershire sauce
- 1 teaspoon lemon juice
- 1/2 teaspoon paprika
- Salt and pepper to taste
- Lettuce leaves, for serving
- Lemon wedges, for garnish

DIRECTIONS

- In a bowl, combine the cooked prawns and diced avocado.
- In another bowl, mix together the Greek yogurt, tomato ketchup, Worcestershire sauce, lemon juice, paprika, salt, and pepper to make the Marie Rose sauce.
- Pour the Marie Rose sauce over the prawn and avocado mixture. Gently toss to coat.
- To serve, arrange lettuce leaves on plates and spoon the prawn and avocado mixture on top.
- Garnish with lemon wedges.
- Serve immediately.

NUTRITIONAL FACTS (PER SERVING)

- Calories: 190kcal
- Total Fat: 9g
- Saturated Fat: 1g
- Trans Fat: 0g
- Cholesterol: 140mg
- Sodium: 430mg
- Carbohydrates: 10g
- Dietary Fiber: 5g
- Sugars: 3g
- Protein: 20g

QUINOA AND ROASTED VEGETABLE STUFFED MUSHROOMS

PREP
15 Mins

COOK
25 Mins

YIELDS
4 Servings

SERVING SIZE
2

INGREDIENTS

- 8 large portobello mushrooms
- 1 cup cooked quinoa
- 1 cup diced mixed vegetables (such as bell peppers, zucchini, carrots)
- 2 cloves garlic, minced
- 1 tablespoon olive oil
- Salt and pepper to taste
- Fresh parsley for garnish (optional)

DIRECTIONS

- Preheat your oven to 375°F (190°C). Clean the mushrooms and remove the stems. Place the mushrooms on a baking sheet lined with parchment paper.
- In a skillet, heat olive oil over medium heat. Add minced garlic and diced vegetables. Sauté until the vegetables are tender, about 5-7 minutes.
- In a bowl, mix the cooked quinoa with the sautéed vegetables. Season with salt and pepper to taste.
- Stuff each mushroom cap with the quinoa and vegetable mixture, pressing it down gently.

NUTRITIONAL FACTS (PER SERVING)

- Calories: 110kcal
- Total Fat: 3g
- Saturated Fat: 0g
- Cholesterol: 0mg
- Sodium: 60mg
- Carbohydrate: 18g
- Dietary Fiber: 3g
- Sugars: 2g
- Protein: 4g

DIRECTIONS

- Bake in the preheated oven for about 20 minutes or until the mushrooms are tender.
- Garnish with fresh parsley if desired, and serve hot.

CURRY-LIME CHICKEN SALAD

PREP	**COOK**	**YIELDS**	**SERVING SIZE**
10 Mins	0 Mins	4 Servings	1/2

INGREDIENTS

- 2 cups cooked chicken breast, shredded or diced
- 1/2 cup non-fat Greek yogurt
- 1 tablespoon lime juice
- 1 teaspoon curry powder
- 1/2 teaspoon ground cumin
- 1/4 teaspoon garlic powder
- Salt and pepper to taste
- 1/4 cup diced celery
- 1/4 cup diced red onion
- 1/4 cup diced bell pepper (any color)
- 2 tablespoons chopped cilantro (optional)

DIRECTIONS

- In a large mixing bowl, combine the shredded or diced chicken breast with non-fat Greek yogurt, lime juice, curry powder, cumin, garlic powder, salt, and pepper. Mix well to combine.
- Add diced celery, red onion, bell pepper, and chopped cilantro (if using) to the chicken mixture. Stir until all ingredients are evenly distributed.
- Taste and adjust seasoning if necessary.
- Serve immediately or chill in the refrigerator for at least 30 minutes before serving to allow flavors to meld.

NUTRITIONAL FACTS (PER SERVING)

- Calories: 120kcal
- Total Fat: 1g
- Saturated Fat: 0g
- Cholesterol: 45mg
- Sodium: 110mg
- Carbohydrates: 3g
- Dietary Fiber: 1g
- Sugars: 1g
- Protein: 22g

SMOKED-TURKEY EGG BITE

PREP	**COOK**	**YIELDS**	**SERVING SIZE**
10 Mins	25 Mins	12 Egg Bites	1

INGREDIENTS

- 4 large eggs
- 1/2 cup fat-free cottage cheese
- 4 oz. smoked turkey breast, diced
- 1/4 cup diced bell peppers (any color)
- 1/4 cup diced onions
- Salt and pepper to taste
- Cooking spray

DIRECTIONS

- Preheat your oven to 350°F (175°C).
- In a blender or food processor, blend eggs and cottage cheese until smooth.
- Stir in diced turkey, bell peppers, onions, salt, and pepper.
- Spray a muffin tin with cooking spray to prevent sticking.
- Pour the egg mixture evenly into the muffin tin, filling each cup about 3/4 full.
- Bake in the preheated oven for 20-25 minutes, or until the egg bites are set and slightly golden on top.
- Allow the egg bites to cool slightly before removing them from the muffin tin.

NUTRITIONAL FACTS (PER SERVING)

- Calories: 40kcal
- Total Fat: 1g
- Saturated Fat: 0.3g
- Cholesterol: 88mg
- Sodium: 160mg
- Carbohydrate: 1g
- Dietary Fiber: 0.2g
- Sugars: 0.6g
- Protein: 7g

DIRECTIONS

- Serve warm and enjoy!

CRUCHY APPLE SALSA

PREP 15 Mins	**COOK** 0 Mins	**YIELDS** 4 Servings	**SERVING SIZE** 1/2

INGREDIENTS

- 2 medium apples, diced (use a mix of sweet and tart varieties for best flavor)
- 1/2 cup diced red onion
- 1/2 cup diced cucumber
- 1/4 cup chopped fresh cilantro
- 1 jalapeño pepper, seeded and finely diced
- Juice of 1 lime
- Salt and pepper to taste

DIRECTIONS

- In a medium bowl, combine diced apples, red onion, cucumber, cilantro, and jalapeño pepper.
- Squeeze lime juice over the mixture and toss to combine.
- Season with salt and pepper to taste.
- Serve immediately or refrigerate until ready to serve.

NUTRITIONAL FACTS
(PER SERVING)

- Calories: 35kcal
- Total Fat: 0g
- Saturated Fat: 0g
- Cholesterol: 0mg
- Sodium: 1mg
- Carbohydrates: 9g
- Dietary Fiber: 2g
- Sugars: 6g
- Protein: 0g

TOFU-GARLIC AIOLI

PREP
10 Mins

COOK
0 Mins

YIELDS
1 Cup

SERVING SIZE
2 Tablespoons

INGREDIENTS

- 1/2 block (about 200g) firm tofu, drained and pressed
- 2 cloves garlic, minced
- 2 tablespoons lemon juice
- 1 tablespoon Dijon mustard
- Salt and pepper to taste
- 1-2 tablespoons water (optional, for desired consistency)
- Fresh herbs (optional, for garnish)

DIRECTIONS

- In a food processor, blend tofu, minced garlic, lemon juice, and Dijon mustard until smooth.
- If the mixture is too thick, add water, one tablespoon at a time, until you reach the desired consistency.
- Season with salt and pepper to taste.
- Garnish with fresh herbs if desired.
- Serve immediately or refrigerate until ready to use.

NUTRITIONAL FACTS
(PER SERVING)

- Calories: 15kcal
- Total Fat: 0.6g
- Saturated Fat: 0.1g
- Cholesterol: 0mg
- Sodium: 25mg
- Carbohydrates: 0.7g
- Dietary Fiber: 0.2g
- Sugars: 0.1g
- Protein: 1.6g

BUFFALO CHICKEN DIP

PREP
10 Mins

COOK
20 Mins

YIELDS
8 Servings

SERVING SIZE
1/4

INGREDIENTS

- 2 cups shredded cooked chicken breast (skinless, boneless)
- 1 cup fat-free Greek yogurt
- 1/4 cup hot sauce (choose a brand with no added sugar)
- 1/4 cup diced celery
- 1/4 cup diced green onions
- 1/4 teaspoon garlic powder
- 1/4 teaspoon onion powder
- Salt and pepper to taste

DIRECTIONS

- Preheat your oven to 350°F (175°C).
- In a mixing bowl, combine shredded chicken, Greek yogurt, hot sauce, diced celery, diced green onions, garlic powder, and onion powder. Mix until well combined.
- Transfer the mixture into a baking dish.
- Bake for 20-25 minutes, or until the dip is hot and bubbly.
- Serve hot with your choice of fresh veggies for dipping.

NUTRITIONAL FACTS (PER SERVING)

- Calories: 55kcal
- Total Fat: 0.3g
- Saturated Fat: 0.1g
- Cholesterol: 18mg
- Sodium: 236mg
- Carbohydrates: 1.2g
- Dietary Fiber: 0.2g
- Total Sugars: 0.8g
- Protein: 10.6g

TOMATO AND MOZZARELLA SALAD WITH BASIL PESTO

PREP	**COOK**	**YIELDS**	**SERVING SIZE**
10 Mins	0 Mins	4 Servings	1/4

INGREDIENTS

- 2 medium tomatoes, sliced
- 4 ounces fresh mozzarella cheese, sliced
- 1/4 cup fresh basil leaves
- 1 tablespoon balsamic vinegar
- Salt and pepper to taste

For the Basil Pesto:

- 1 cup fresh basil leaves
- 2 cloves garlic
- 2 tablespoons lemon juice
- 2 tablespoons water
- Salt and pepper to taste

DIRECTIONS

- In a large mixing bowl, combine chopped endives, walnuts, and crumbled Roquefort cheese.
- Drizzle lemon juice over the salad and toss gently to combine.
- Season with salt and pepper to taste.
- Serve immediately.

NUTRITIONAL FACTS (PER SERVING)

- Calories: 90kcal
- Total Fat: 7g
- Saturated Fat: 2g
- Cholesterol: 6mg
- Sodium: 220mg
- Carbohydrates: 4g
- Dietary Fiber: 2g
- Sugars: 1g
- Protein: 4g

HONEYDEW AND MINT GRANITA

PREP
15 Mins | **COOK**
0 Mins | **YIELDS**
6 Servings | **SERVING SIZE**
1/2

INGREDIENTS

- 1 large honeydew melon, peeled, seeded, and chopped
- 1/4 cup fresh mint leaves
- 1 tablespoon fresh lime juice
- Optional: sweetener (such as stevia or monk fruit sweetener) to taste

DIRECTIONS

- In a blender or food processor, combine the chopped honeydew melon, fresh mint leaves, and lime juice.
- Blend until smooth.
- Taste the mixture and add sweetener if desired, blending again to incorporate.
- Pour the mixture into a shallow dish or baking pan.
- Place the dish in the freezer.
- After 1 hour, use a fork to scrape and fluff the partially frozen mixture.
- Return the dish to the freezer and repeat the scraping process every 30 minutes until the granita is fully frozen and fluffy, about 2-3 hours total.

**NUTRITIONAL FACTS
(PER SERVING)**

- Calories: 40kcal
- Total Fat: 0g
- Saturated Fat: 0g
- Cholesterol: 0mg
- Sodium: 25mg
- Carbohydrate: 10g
- Dietary Fiber: 1g
- Sugars: 9g
- Protein: 1g

DIRECTIONS

- Serve the granita immediately or transfer it to an airtight container and store it in the freezer until ready to serve.

TOMATO AND RED ONION SALSA

PREP	**COOK**	**YIELDS**	**SERVING SIZE**
10 Mins	0 Mins	4 Servings	1/2

INGREDIENTS

- 3 large tomatoes, diced
- 1 small red onion, finely diced
- 1/4 cup fresh cilantro, chopped
- 2 tablespoons lime juice
- 1 jalapeño pepper, seeded and minced (optional for added heat)
- Salt and pepper to taste

DIRECTIONS

- In a mixing bowl, combine diced tomatoes, finely diced red onion, chopped cilantro, lime juice, and minced jalapeño pepper (if using).
- Season with salt and pepper to taste.
- Mix well until all ingredients are evenly distributed.

NUTRITIONAL FACTS (PER SERVING)

- Calories: 25kcal
- Total Fat: 0g
- Saturated Fat: 0g
- Cholesterol: 0mg
- Sodium: 5mg
- Carbohydrates: 6g
- Dietary Fiber: 1g
- Sugars: 3g
- Protein: 1g

THAI BEEF SALAD WITH LIME DRESSING AND PEANUTS

PREP 10 Mins | **COOK** 6 Mins | **YIELDS** 4 Servings | **SERVING SIZE** 1/4

INGREDIENTS

- 1 lb lean beef (such as sirloin or flank steak), sliced thinly
- 4 cups mixed salad greens (e.g., lettuce, spinach, arugula)
- 1 cup cucumber, thinly sliced
- 1 cup cherry tomatoes, halved
- 1/4 cup red onion, thinly sliced
- 1/4 cup fresh cilantro, chopped
- 2 tbsp peanuts, crushed (unsalted)
- 1 lime, juiced
- 1 tbsp fish sauce
- 1 tbsp soy sauce (low sodium)
- 1 clove garlic, minced
- 1 tsp ginger, grated
- Salt and pepper to taste

DIRECTIONS

- In a bowl, combine lime juice, fish sauce, soy sauce, garlic, ginger, and optional chili peppers. Add the sliced beef and let it marinate for at least 15 minutes.
- Prepare the Salad: In a large bowl, toss together the mixed salad greens, cucumber, cherry tomatoes, red onion, and cilantro.
- Cook the Beef: Heat a non-stick skillet over medium-high heat. Add the marinated beef slices and cook for 2-3 minutes on each side until cooked through. Remove from heat and let it rest for a few minutes.
- Assemble the Salad: Arrange the cooked beef slices on top of the prepared salad.

NUTRITIONAL FACTS (PER SERVING)

- Calories: 220kcal
- Protein: 25g
- Carbohydrates: 8g
- Fat: 10g
- Fiber: 2g
- Sugar: 3g
- Sodium: 400mg

DIRECTIONS

- Make the Dressing: In a small bowl, whisk together any remaining marinade with additional lime juice if desired.
- Serve: Drizzle the dressing over the salad and sprinkle with crushed peanuts.

CHIA SEED PUDDING WITH MIXED BERRIES AND COCONUT

PREP
5 Mins

COOK
0 Mins

YIELDS
2 Servings

SERVING SIZE
1/2

INGREDIENTS

- 1/4 cup chia seeds
- 1 cup unsweetened almond milk (or any other unsweetened plant-based milk)
- 1/2 teaspoon vanilla extract
- 1/2 cup mixed berries (such as strawberries, blueberries, raspberries)
- 1 tablespoon unsweetened shredded coconut

DIRECTIONS

- In a mixing bowl, combine chia seeds, almond milk, and vanilla extract. Stir well.
- Let the mixture sit for about 5 minutes, then stir again to break up any clumps of chia seeds.
- Cover the bowl and refrigerate for at least 2 hours or overnight, until the mixture thickens into a pudding-like consistency.
- Before serving, divide the chia seed pudding into serving bowls.
- Top each serving with mixed berries and sprinkle with shredded coconut.

NUTRITIONAL FACTS (PER SERVING)

- Calories: 90kcal
- Total Fat: 5g
- Saturated Fat: 1g
- Cholesterol: 0mg
- Sodium: 80mg
- Carbohydrates: 8g
- Dietary Fiber: 6g
- Sugars: 1g
- Protein: 4g

PEA, LEEK AND MINT SOUP

PREP
10 Mins

COOK
15 Mins

YIELDS
4 Servings

SERVING SIZE
1

INGREDIENTS

- 1 medium leek, sliced
- 3 cups frozen peas
- 3 cups vegetable broth
- 1 tablespoon fresh mint leaves
- Salt and pepper to taste

DIRECTIONS

- In a large pot, add sliced leeks and a splash of vegetable broth. Sauté over medium heat until leeks are softened, about 5 minutes.
- Add frozen peas and remaining vegetable broth to the pot. Bring to a simmer and cook for 5-7 minutes until peas are tender.
- Remove the pot from heat and stir in fresh mint leaves.
- Using an immersion blender or transferring to a blender in batches, blend the soup until smooth.
- Season with salt and pepper to taste.
- Serve hot, garnished with additional fresh mint leaves if desired.

NUTRITIONAL FACTS (PER SERVING)

- Calories: 85kcal
- Total Fat: 0.6g
- Saturated Fat: 0.1g
- Cholesterol: 0mg
- Sodium: 372mg
- Carbohydrate: 14.8g
- Dietary Fiber: 5.5g
- Sugars: 5.3g
- Protein: 5.3g

PUMPKIN SOUP

PREP 10 Mins	**COOK** 20 Mins	**YIELDS** 6 Servings	**SERVING SIZE** 1

INGREDIENTS

- 1 can (15 oz) pumpkin puree (not pumpkin pie filling)
- 4 cups low-sodium chicken or vegetable broth
- 1 small onion, diced
- 2 cloves garlic, minced
- 1 teaspoon ground ginger
- 1 teaspoon ground cinnamon
- 1/4 teaspoon ground nutmeg
- Salt and pepper to taste
- Optional toppings: chopped fresh parsley, plain non-fat Greek yogurt

DIRECTIONS

- In a large pot, sauté diced onion and minced garlic over medium heat until softened, about 3-4 minutes.
- Add pumpkin puree, chicken or vegetable broth, ground ginger, ground cinnamon, and ground nutmeg to the pot. Stir well to combine.
- Bring the mixture to a simmer and let it cook for about 15-20 minutes, stirring occasionally.
- Once the soup is heated through and flavors have melded together, remove from heat. Season with salt and pepper to taste.
- Using an immersion blender or transferring the soup in batches to a regular blender, blend until smooth and creamy.

**NUTRITIONAL FACTS
(PER SERVING)**

- Calories: 50kcal
- Total Fat: 0g
- Saturated Fat: 0g
- Cholesterol: 0mg
- Sodium: 100mg
- Carbohydrates: 10g
- Dietary Fiber: 3g
- Sugars: 4g
- Protein: 2g

DIRECTIONS

- Serve hot, optionally garnished with chopped fresh parsley or a dollop of plain non-fat Greek yogurt.

TEXAS CAVIAR

PREP
15 Mins

COOK
0 Mins

YIELDS
8 Servings

SERVING SIZE
1/2

INGREDIENTS

- 1 can (15 ounces) black beans, drained and rinsed
- 1 can (15 ounces) black-eyed peas, drained and rinsed
- 1 can (15 ounces) corn, drained
- 1 medium red bell pepper, diced
- 1 medium green bell pepper, diced
- 1 small red onion, diced
- 1 jalapeño pepper, seeded and minced (optional for spice)
- 1/4 cup chopped fresh cilantro
- 1/4 cup lime juice (about 2 limes)
- 2 tablespoons apple cider vinegar
- Salt and pepper to taste

DIRECTIONS

- In a large mixing bowl, combine the black beans, black-eyed peas, corn, diced bell peppers, diced onion, minced jalapeño (if using), and chopped cilantro.
- In a small bowl, whisk together the lime juice and apple cider vinegar. Pour the dressing over the bean mixture and toss until well combined.
- Season with salt and pepper to taste.
- Cover and refrigerate for at least 1 hour to allow the flavors to meld.
- Serve chilled.

NUTRITIONAL FACTS (PER SERVING)

- Calories: 120kcal
- Total Fat: 0.5g
- Saturated Fat: 0g
- Cholesterol: 0mg
- Sodium: 240mg
- Carbohydrates: 24g
- Dietary Fiber: 5g
- Total Sugars: 4g
- Protein: 6g

SMOKED MACKEREL SALAD WITH APPLE AND HORSERADISH DRESSING

PREP	**COOK**	**YIELDS**	**SERVING SIZE**
10 Mins	0 Mins	2 Servings	2

INGREDIENTS

- 200g smoked mackerel fillets, skin removed
- 1 apple, thinly sliced
- 1 small red onion, thinly sliced
- 2 cups mixed salad greens (e.g., spinach, arugula, lettuce)
- 2 tablespoons fat-free Greek yogurt
- 1 tablespoon prepared horseradish
- 1 tablespoon lemon juice
- Salt and pepper to taste

DIRECTIONS

- In a small bowl, mix together the fat-free Greek yogurt, prepared horseradish, lemon juice, salt, and pepper to make the dressing. Adjust seasoning to taste.
- In a large mixing bowl, combine the sliced apple, sliced red onion, and mixed salad greens.
- Break the smoked mackerel fillets into bite-sized pieces and add them to the salad mixture.
- Drizzle the prepared dressing over the salad and toss gently to combine.
- Divide the salad evenly between two plates or bowls.
- Serve immediately and enjoy!

NUTRITIONAL FACTS (PER SERVING)

- Calories: 160kcal
- Total Fat: 5g
- Saturated Fat: 1g
- Cholesterol: 30mg
- Sodium: 330mg
- Carbohydrates: 12g
- Dietary Fiber: 3g
- Sugars: 7g
- Protein: 18g

KOHLRABI AND CARROT SLAW WITH LEMON DRESSING

PREP	**COOK**	**YIELDS**	**SERVING SIZE**
15 Mins	0 Mins	4 Servings	1

INGREDIENTS

- 2 kohlrabi bulbs, peeled and grated
- 2 large carrots, peeled and grated
- 1/4 cup fresh parsley, chopped
- 1 tablespoon lemon zest
- 2 tablespoons lemon juice
- 1 teaspoon Dijon mustard
- Salt and pepper to taste

DIRECTIONS

- In a large bowl, combine the grated kohlrabi, grated carrots, chopped parsley, and lemon zest.
- In a small bowl, whisk together the lemon juice, Dijon mustard, salt, and pepper until well combined.
- Pour the lemon dressing over the kohlrabi and carrot mixture and toss until everything is evenly coated.
- Taste and adjust seasoning if necessary.
- Refrigerate for at least 30 minutes before serving to allow the flavors to meld together.

NUTRITIONAL FACTS
(PER SERVING)

- Calories: 45kcal
- Total Fat: 0g
- Saturated Fat: 0g
- Cholesterol: 0mg
- Sodium: 70mg
- Carbohydrates: 10g
- Dietary Fiber: 4g
- Sugars: 4g
- Protein: 2g

PEACHY KEEN SMOOTHIE

PREP 5 Mins	**COOK** 0 Mins	**YIELDS** 2 Servings	**SERVING SIZE** 1/2

INGREDIENTS

- 1 cup frozen peaches (unsweetened)
- 1/2 cup non-fat Greek yogurt
- 1/2 cup unsweetened almond milk (or any other milk of your choice)
- 1/4 teaspoon vanilla extract
- 1/4 teaspoon ground cinnamon
- 1/2 cup ice cubes

DIRECTIONS

- Place all the ingredients into a blender.
- Blend until smooth and creamy.
- Pour into glasses and serve immediately.

NUTRITIONAL FACTS (PER SERVING)

- Calories: 70kcal
- Total Fat: 0g
- Saturated Fat: 0g
- Cholesterol: 0mg
- Sodium: 45mg
- Carbohydrates: 12g
- Dietary Fiber: 2g
- Sugars: 9g
- Protein: 6g

RASPBERRY COCONUT SMOOTHIE

PREP
5 Mins

COOK
0 Mins

YIELDS
2 Servings

SERVING SIZE
1/2

INGREDIENTS

- 1 cup unsweetened coconut milk
- 1 cup frozen raspberries
- 1/2 cup unsweetened shredded coconut
- 1/2 teaspoon vanilla extract
- 1/2 cup ice cubes

DIRECTIONS

- Combine all ingredients in a blender.
- Blend until smooth and creamy.
- Pour into glasses and serve immediately.

NUTRITIONAL FACTS (PER SERVING)

- Calories: 70kcal
- Total Fat: 4g
- Saturated Fat: 3g
- Cholesterol: 0mg
- Sodium: 25mg
- Carbohydrates: 8g
- Dietary Fiber: 4g
- Sugars: 3g
- Protein: 1g

Meal plan

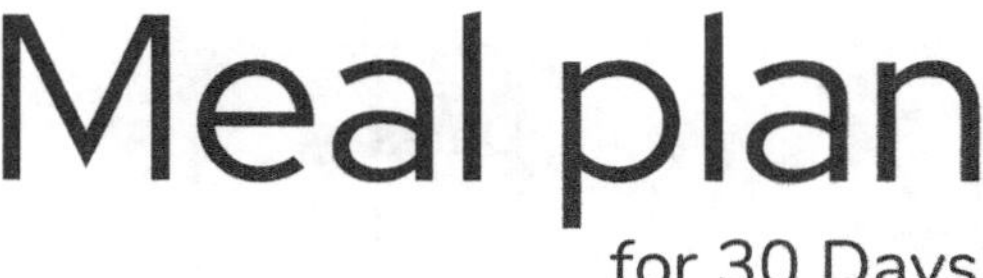

for 30 Days

Dates

____

	BREAKFAST	LUNCH	DINNER
MON	Veggie Omelette	Mexican Salad with Black Beans, Corn, and Avocado	Grilled Salmon with Steamed Broccoli
TUE	Greek Yogurt Parfait with Berries	Turkey Lettuce Wraps	Quinoa-Stuffed Bell Peppers
WED	Spanish Omelette (Tortilla Española)	Greek Salad with Feta Cheese	Ratatouille
THU	Overnight Oats with Chia Seeds and Fruit	Italian Caprese Salad	Baked Cod with Roasted Vegetables
FRI	Miso Soup with Tofu and Seaweed	Sushi Rolls with Vegetable Fillings	Stir-Fried Tofu with Vegetables
SAT	Chinese Congee with Pickled Vegetables	Vietnamese Fresh Spring Rolls	Thai Green Curry with Tofu and Vegetables

Meal plan

for 30 Days

Dates

____

	BREAKFAST	LUNCH	DINNER
SUN	Whole grain toast with mashed avocado and sliced tomato	Egg salad stuffed in bell pepper halves served with a side of carrot sticks	Grilled steak with roasted green beans and a side of quinoa

Week 2-4

- Continue to repeat and vary these meal ideas throughout the 30-day period, incorporating a wide range of fruits, vegetables, lean proteins, and whole grains. Remember to drink plenty of water throughout the day and listen to your body's hunger and fullness cues.

ZERO POINT FOOD LIST

Zero Point Fruits

- Apples
- Apricots
- Bananas
- Blackberries
- Blueberries
- Cantaloupe
- Cherries
- Clementine
- Coconut
- Cranberries
- Dates
- Dragon Fruit
- Figs
- Grapefruit
- Grapes (any variety)
- Guava
- Honeydew Melon
- Jackfruit
- Kiwi
- Lemon
- Lime
- Mango
- Oranges
- Passion Fruit
- Peach
- Pears
- Pineapple
- Plums
- Pomegranates
- Raspberries
- Starfruit
- Strawberries
- Watermelon

BEANS & LEGUMES

- Adzuki beans
- Alfalfa sprouts
- Bean sprouts
- Black beans
- Black-eyed peas
- Cannellini beans
- Chickpeas
- Edamame
- Fava beans
- Great Northern beans
- Hominy
- Kidney beans
- Lentils
- Lima beans
- Lupini beans
- Navy beans
- Pinto beans
- Refried beans, canned, fat-free
- Soy beans

CHICKEN & TURKEY BREAST

- Ground chicken breast
- Ground turkey, 98% fat-free
- Ground turkey breast
- Skinless chicken breast
- Skinless turkey breast

EGGS

- Egg substitute
- Egg whites
- Egg yolks
- Eggs

**Zero Point Vegetables
(Starchy & Non-Starchy)**

- Arrowroot, raw
- Artichoke
- Arugula
- Asparagus
- Broccoli
- Beans (black, adzuki, cannellini, garbanzo, kidney, great northern, lima, pinto, etc.)
- Beans, refried (canned, fat-free, no added sugar)
- Green Beans
- Bok Choy
- Brussel Sprouts
- Cabbage
- Carrots
- Cauliflower
- Celery
- Chard
- Chickpeas
- Collards
- Corn
- Cucumber
- Daikon
- Edamame
- Eggplant
- Endive
- Fennel
- Ginger Root
- Kale
- Leeks
- Lettuce (any variety)
- Mushrooms
- Okra
- Peas
- Peppers (bell)
- Pickles (without sugar)
- Pumpkin
- Radishes
- Scallions (green onions)
- Spinach
- Sprouts
- Squash
- Tomatoes
- Turnips
- Zucchini

Zero Point Herbs and Spices

- Basil
- Chives
- Cinnamon
- Dill Weed
- Garlic
- Garlic Salt
- Italian Seasoning
- Oregano
- Paprika
- Parsley
- Pepper
- Peppermint
- Pumpkin Spice
- Rosemary
- Sage
- Salt
- Thyme

Zero Point Meat, Seafood and Poultry

- Calamari, grilled
- Chicken Breast (boneless, skinless)
- Crab (Alasaka king, Dungeness, queen, king)
- Crayfish
- Eggs
- Bass Fish
- Bluefish
- Carp
- Catfish
- Cod
- Eel
- Grouper
- Haddock
- Halibut
- Lobster
- Mackerel Fish
- Mussels
- Octopus
- Oysters
- Salmon (Atlantic and farm raised)
- Sardines
- Sea Bass
- Shrimp
- Sturgeon Fish
- Swordfish
- Tilapia Fish
- Tuna (canned in water, drained)
- Tofu
- Trout (rainbow)
- Turkey breast (ground, tenderloin, etc. 99% fat-free)

FISH/SHELLFISH

- Abalone
- Alaskan king crab
- Anchovies, in water
- Arctic char
- Bluefish
- Branzino
- Butterfish
- Canned tuna, in water
- Carp
- Catfish
- Caviar
- Clams
- Cod
- Crabmeat, lump
- Crayfish
- Cuttlefish
- Dungeness crab
- Eel
- Fish roe
- Flounder
- Grouper
- Haddock
- Halibut
- Herring
- Lobster
- Mahi mahi
- Monkfish
- Mussels
- Octopus
- Orange roughy
- Oysters
- Perch
- Pike
- Pollock
- Pompano
- Salmon
- Sardines, canned in water or sauce
- Sashimi
- Scallops
- Sea bass
- Sea cucumber
- Sea urchin
- Shrimp
- Smelt
- Smoked haddock
- Smoked salmon
- Smoked sturgeon
- Smoked trout
- Smoked whitefish
- Snails
- Snapper
- Sole
- Squid

- Steelhead trout
- Striped bass
- Sturgeon
- Swordfish
- Tilapia
- Trout
- Tuna
- Turbot
- Wahoo
- Whitefish

Zero Point Drinks

- Water
- Coffee, black (without sugar)
- Coke Zero (all varieties)
- Diet Coke (all varieties)
- Fresca (all varieties)
- Gatorade Zero
- Sparkling Ice Water (all flavors) etc.

- **Zero Point Snacks**
- Applesauce, unsweetened
- Fruit cup (canned in water pack, no sugar added)
- Fruit cup (fresh)
- Vegetable Sticks
- Yogurt (greek, plain, fat-free, unsweetened)

IMPORTANT NOTICE!!!

We chose to make costs low so it can be accessible to everyone who would love to lose weight. As a result, we didn't include pictures for each recipes.

Please, reach out to us at **popoolaadenike805@gmail.com** if you would like to receive the pictures for each recipes.

HAPPY COOKING!

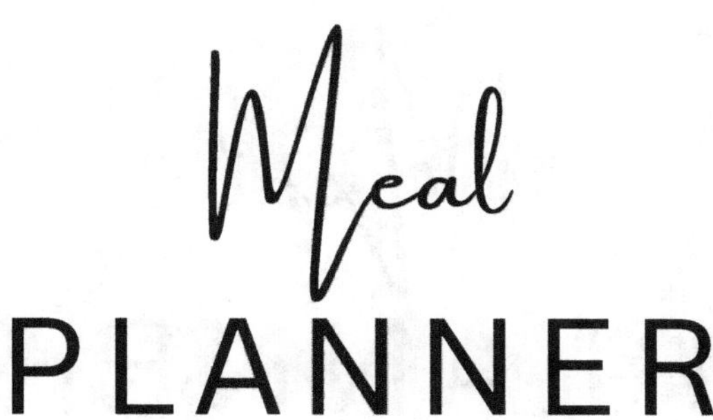

Meal PLANNER

WEEK :

DATE :

MONDAY

B

L

D

S

TUESDAY

B

L

D

S

WEDNESDAY

B

L

D

S

THURSDAY

B

L

D

S

FRIDAY

B

L

D

S

SATURDAY

B

L

D

S

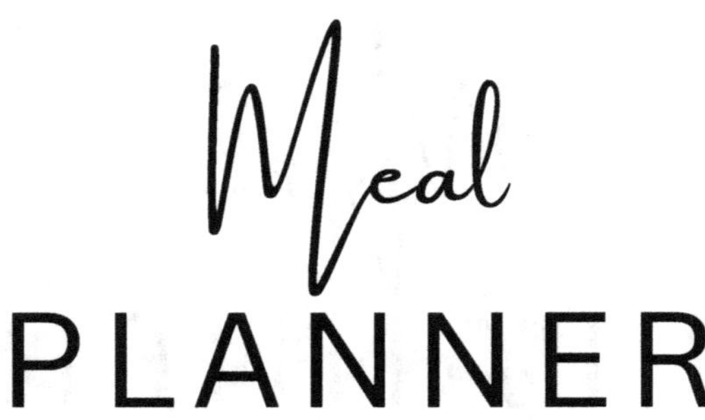

Meal PLANNER

WEEK :

DATE :

MONDAY

B

L

D

S

THURSDAY

B

L

D

S

TUESDAY

B

L

D

S

FRIDAY

B

L

D

S

WEDNESDAY

B

L

D

S

SATURDAY

B

L

D

S

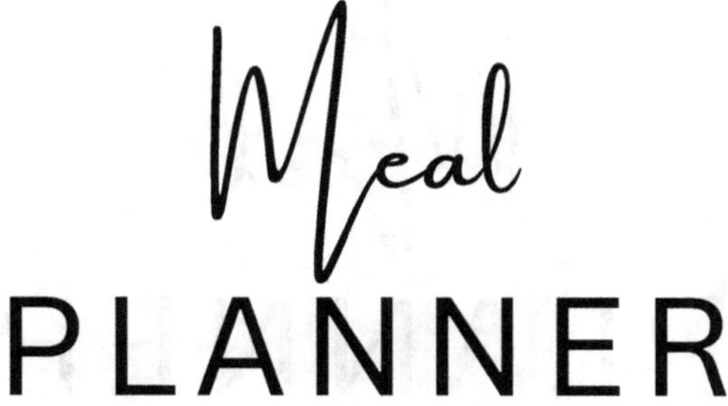

PLANNER

WEEK :

DATE :

MONDAY

B

L

D

S

TUESDAY

B

L

D

S

WEDNESDAY

B

L

D

S

THURSDAY

B

L

D

S

FRIDAY

B

L

D

S

SATURDAY

B

L

D

S

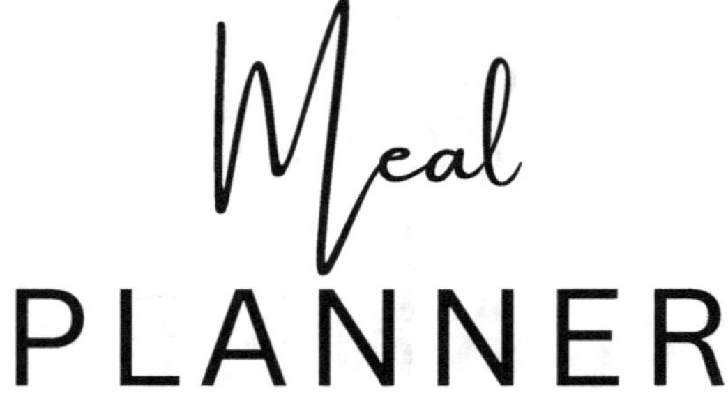

PLANNER

WEEK :

DATE :

MONDAY

B

L

D

S

TUESDAY

B

L

D

S

WEDNESDAY

B

L

D

S

THURSDAY

B

L

D

S

FRIDAY

B

L

D

S

SATURDAY

B

L

D

S

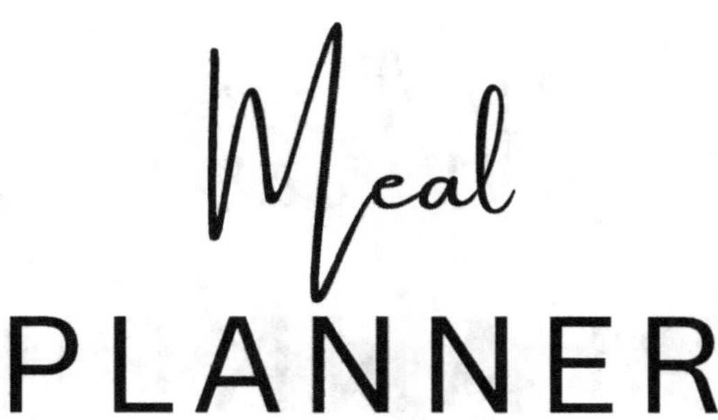

PLANNER

WEEK :

DATE :

MONDAY

B

L

D

S

TUESDAY

B

L

D

S

WEDNESDAY

B

L

D

S

THURSDAY

B

L

D

S

FRIDAY

B

L

D

S

SATURDAY

B

L

D

S

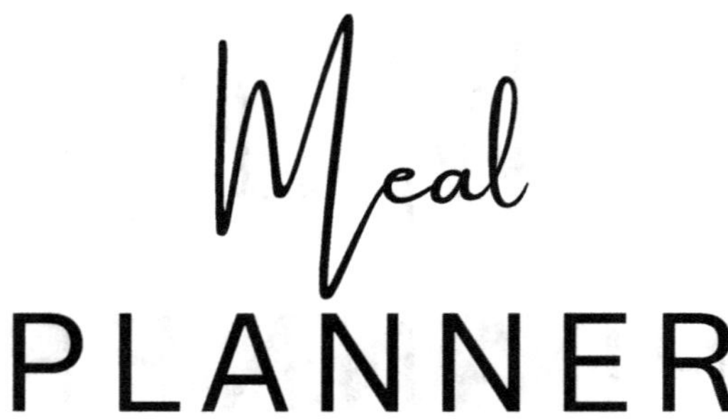

PLANNER

WEEK :

DATE :

MONDAY

B

L

D

S

TUESDAY

B

L

D

S

WEDNESDAY

B

L

D

S

THURSDAY

B

L

D

S

FRIDAY

B

L

D

S

SATURDAY

B

L

D

S